This book was written in an effort to help adoptive & foster families by portraying the concerns and triumphs of fictitious characters designed to promote social understanding and mental well being.

A MONSTER GOT ME !

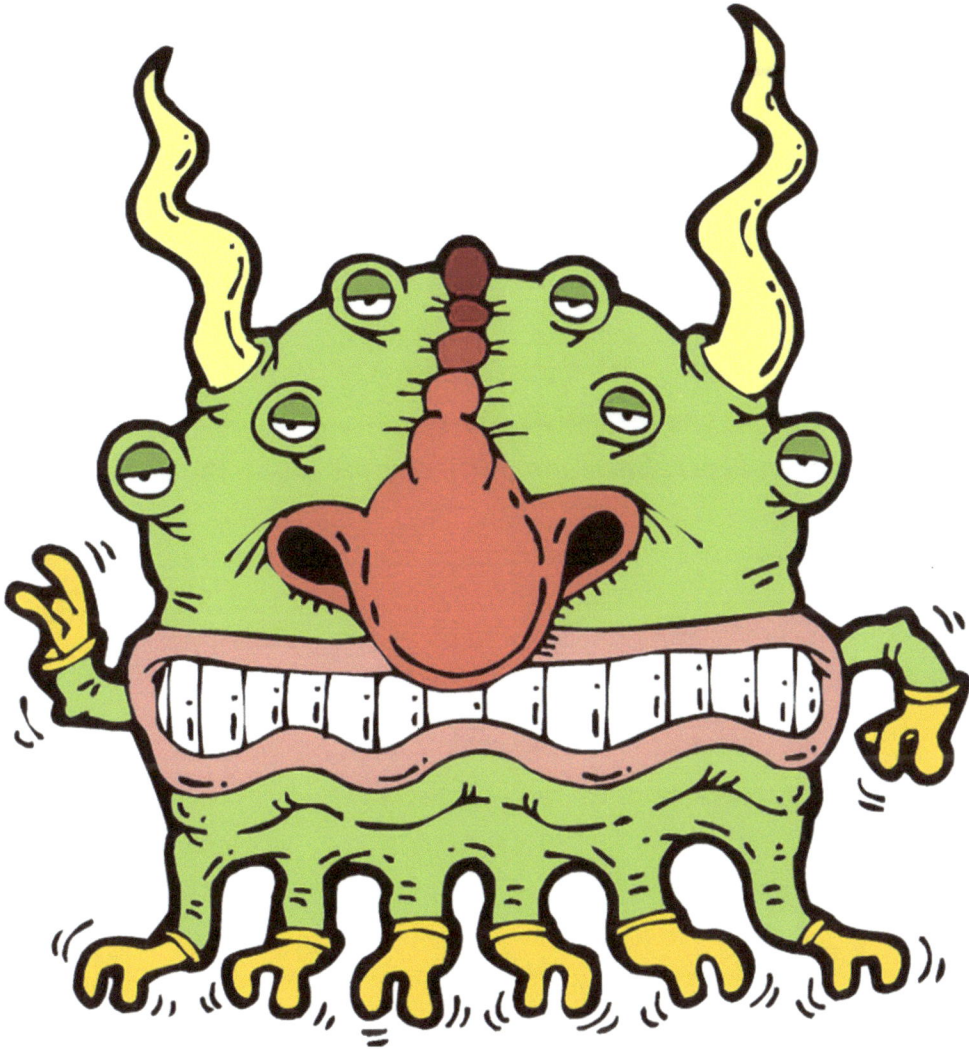

By
Charles Joseph Stippick

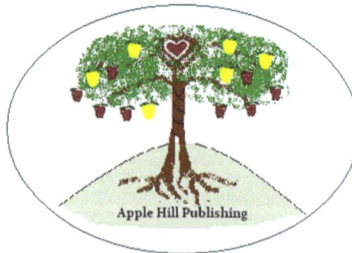

Apple Hill Publishing

applehillpublishing.com

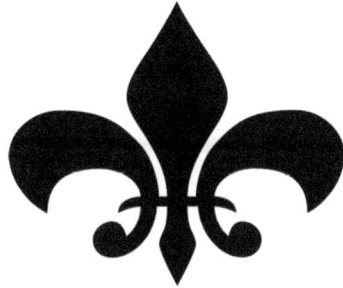

All characters in this book are fictional. Any resemblance to anyone living or dead is coincidental. In addition, it is not meant for any parts of this story to be recreated or to be mimicked. The stories and situations told in this book are metaphors to be used only as examples and not to be recreated in any way shape or form. Please discuss this with your child and make sure that they understand that this story is fiction. The publisher and author are not responsible for anyone reenacting any portion of this book.

A PREFACE IN THE FORM OF A POEM

One Child's View

I see the world through tired eyes.

I feel angry and despise of things that happened because of my size.

I see the world through tired eyes.

People tend to criticize when I need to tell them lies to avoid the pain and inward cries.

I see the world through tired eyes.

I feel old and wise beyond my years and hope one day you will set aside your fears;
And realize through all the tears, that all I need is to love and understand myself.

I see the world through tired eyes.

Don't give up on me, something bad happened and left the scar that you see!
Forgive, be patient and kind, for my world is new, and I'm not yet sure about you.

I see the world through tired eyes.

If you don't give up on me, I won't give up on you.

-Charles J. Stippick

This book is dedicated to Families.

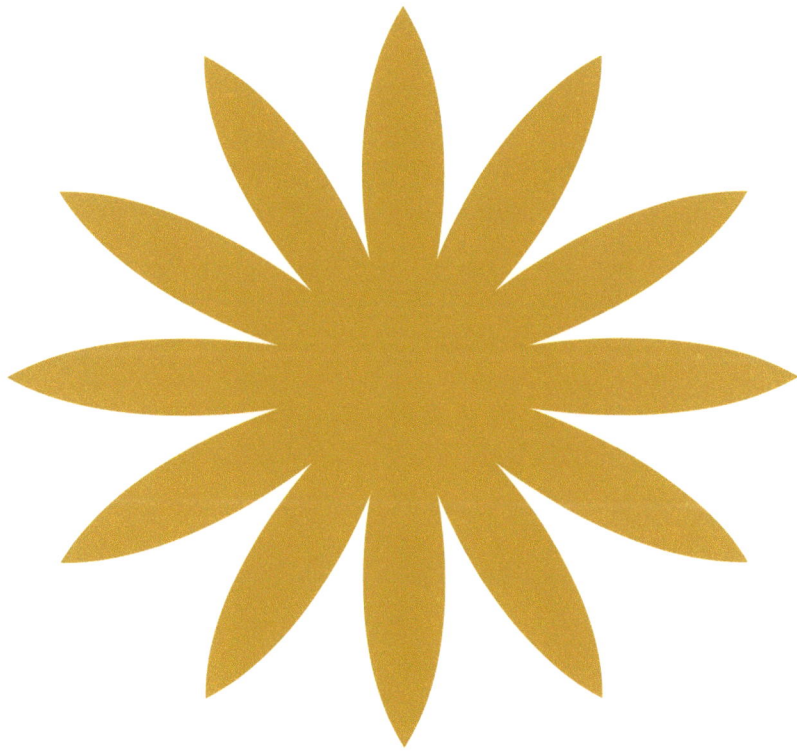

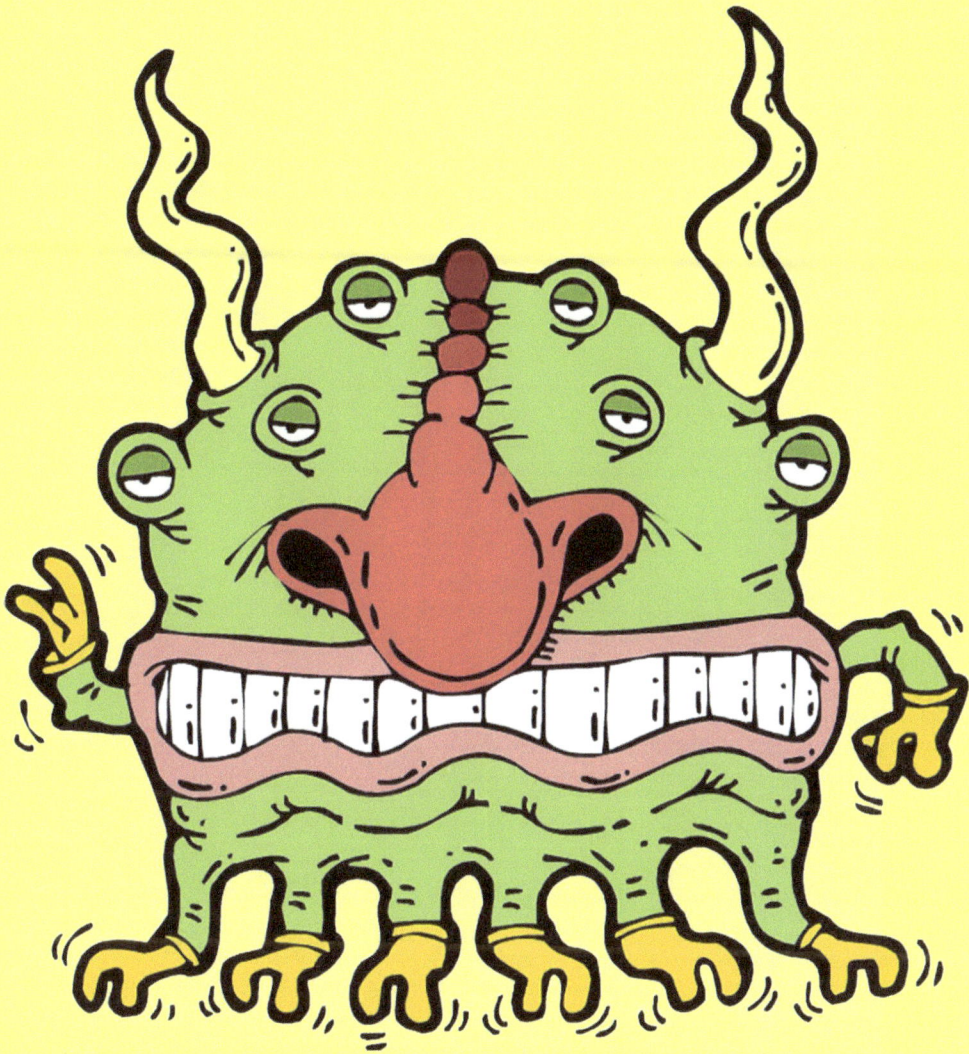

A monster got me, this is true.

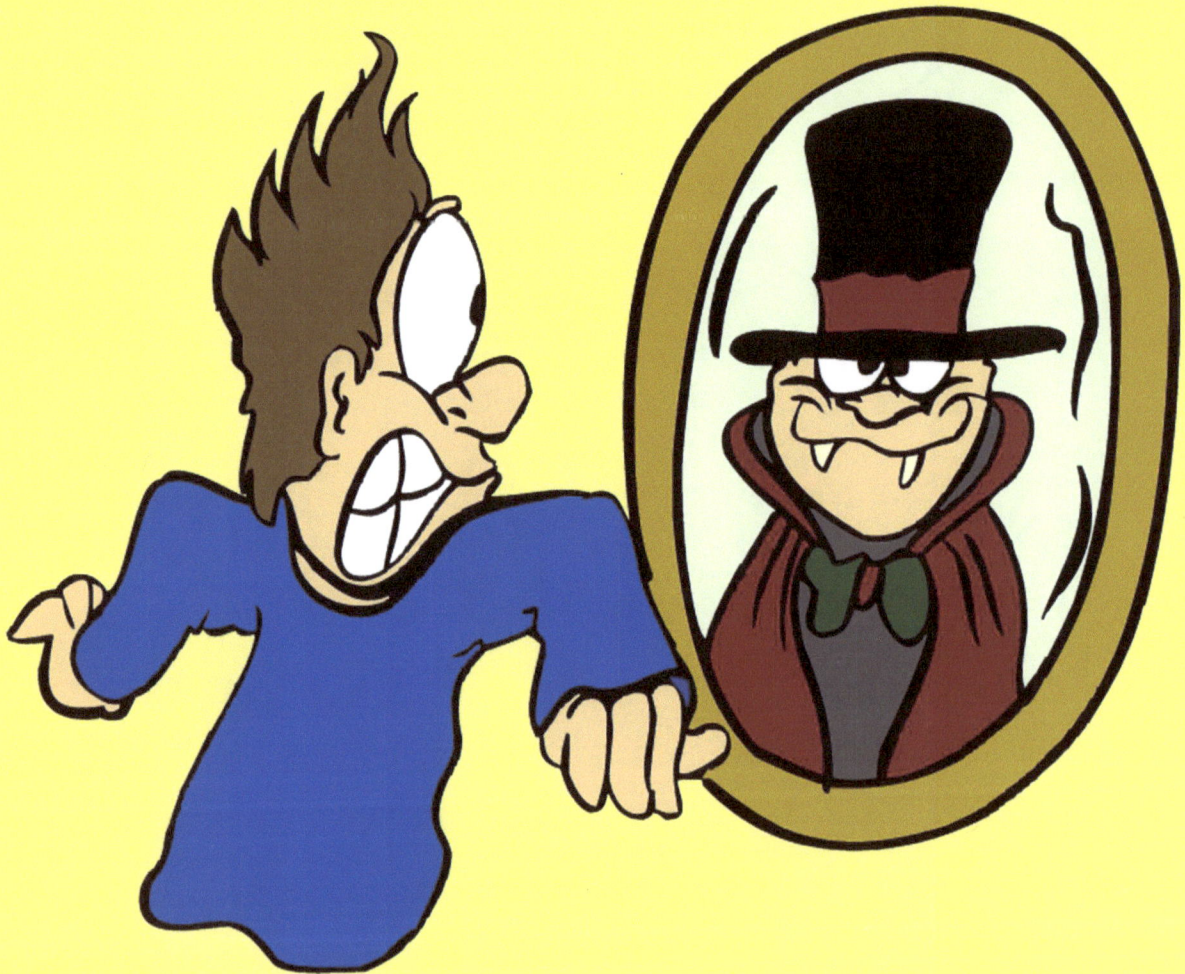

It looked like me.

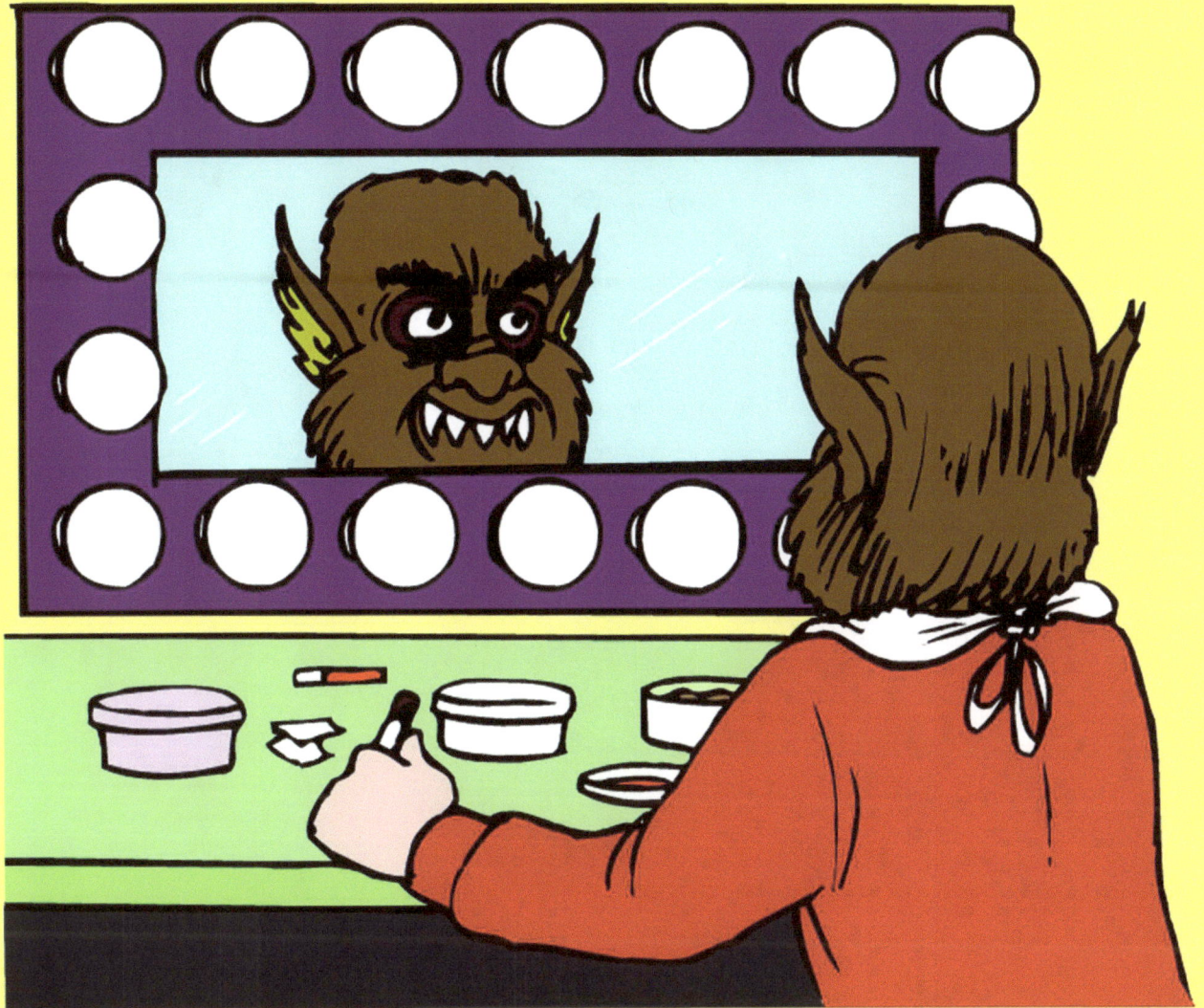

It looked like you.

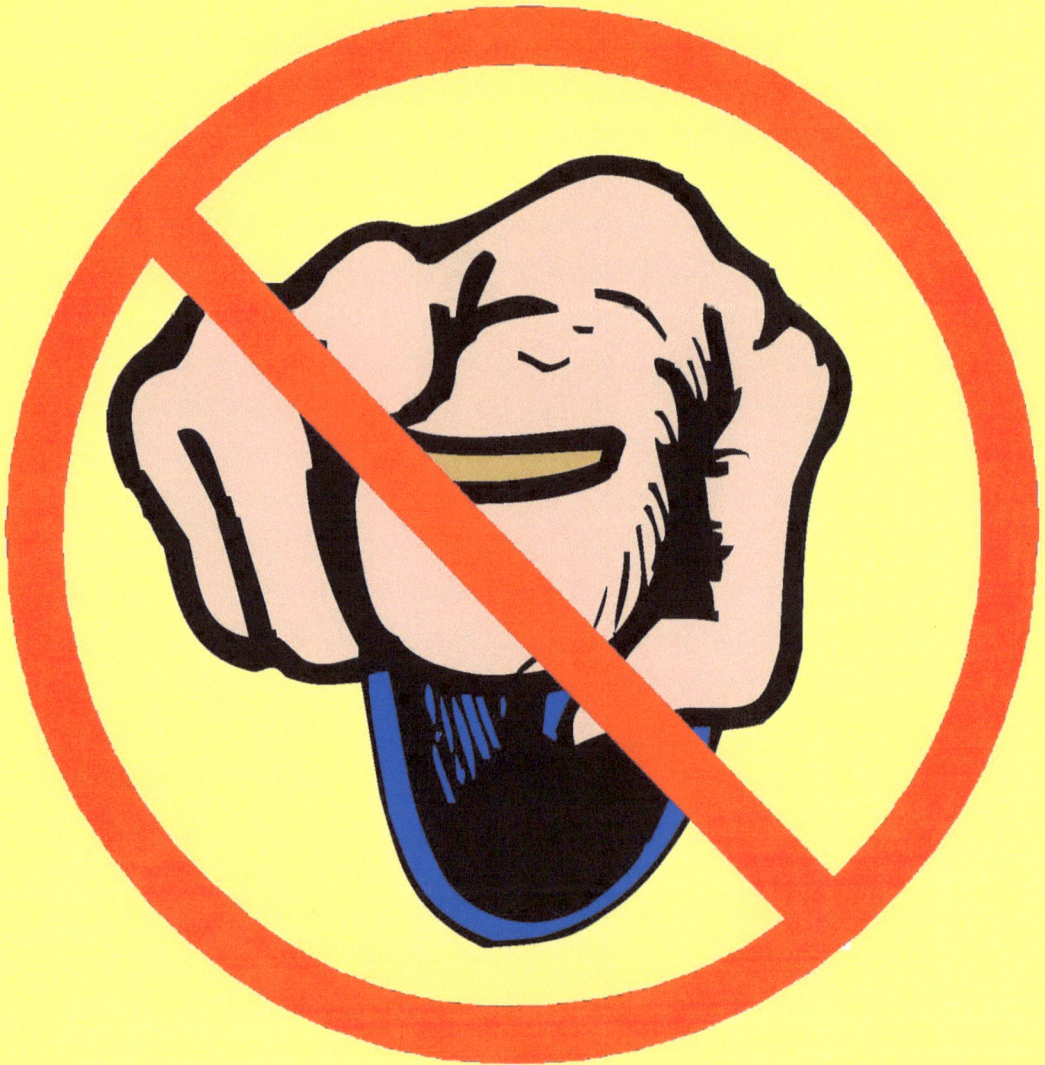

A monster got me,
was not my fault.

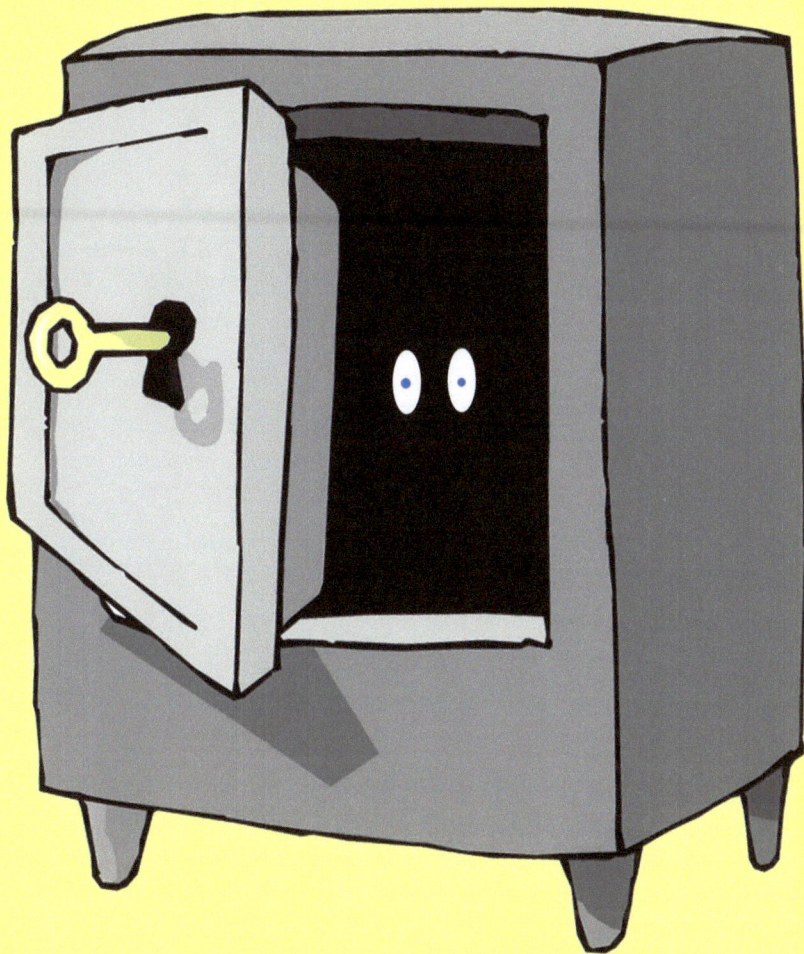

I do not live in an iron vault.

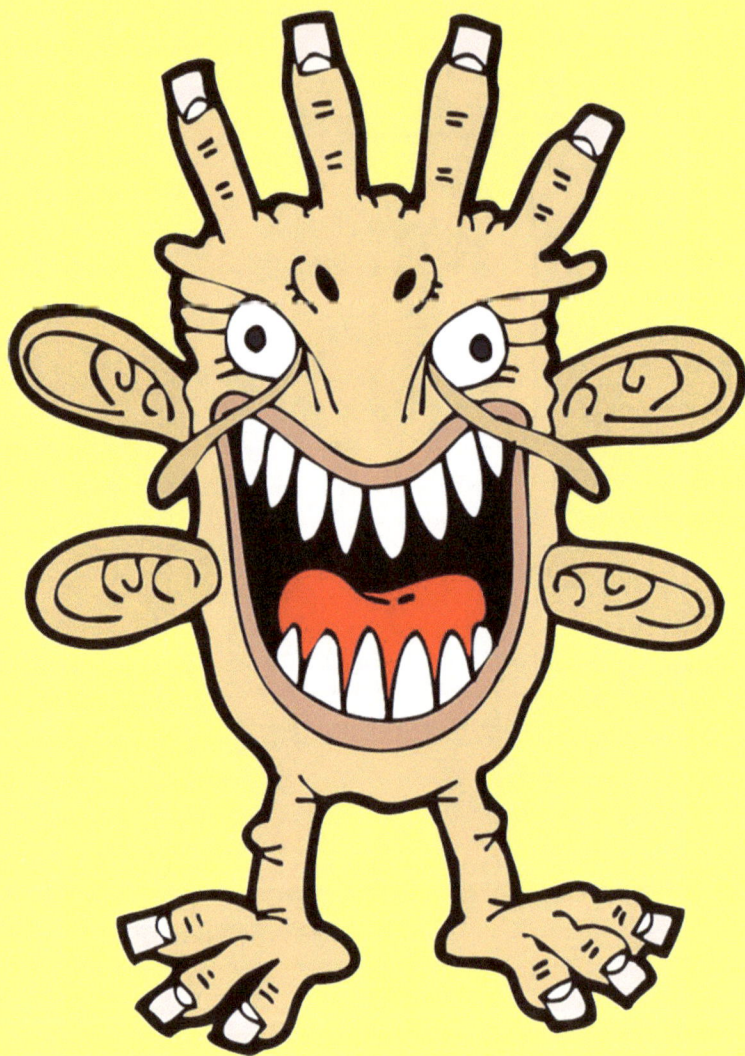

A monster got me this is true.

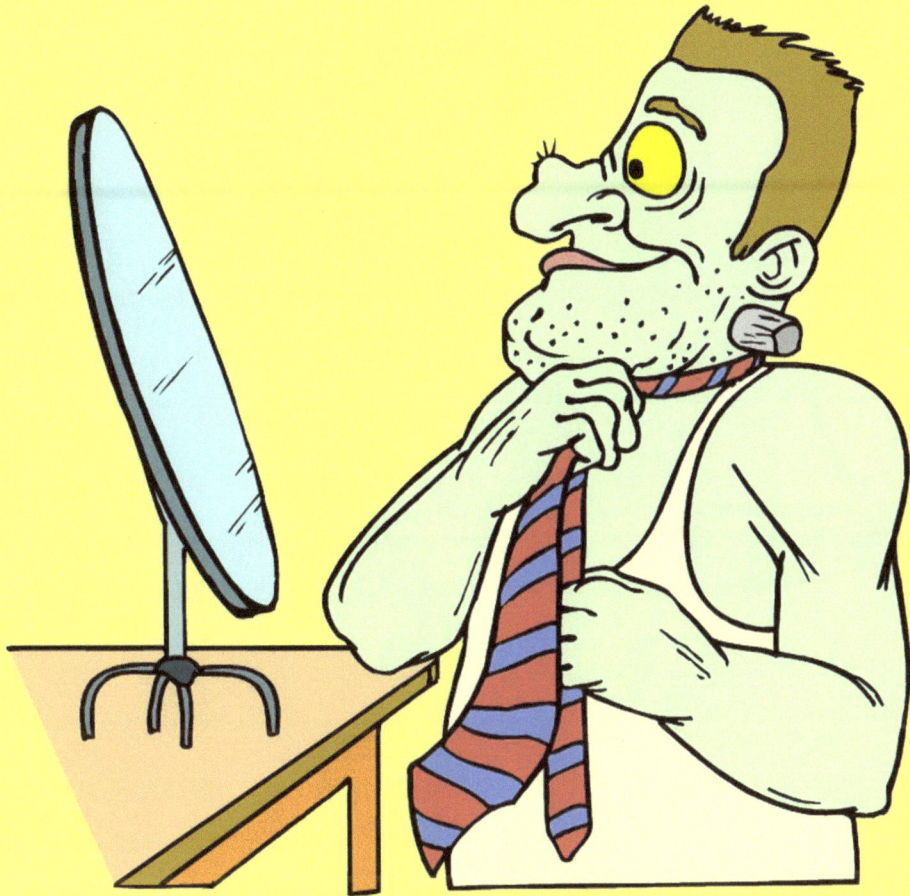

It looked like me.

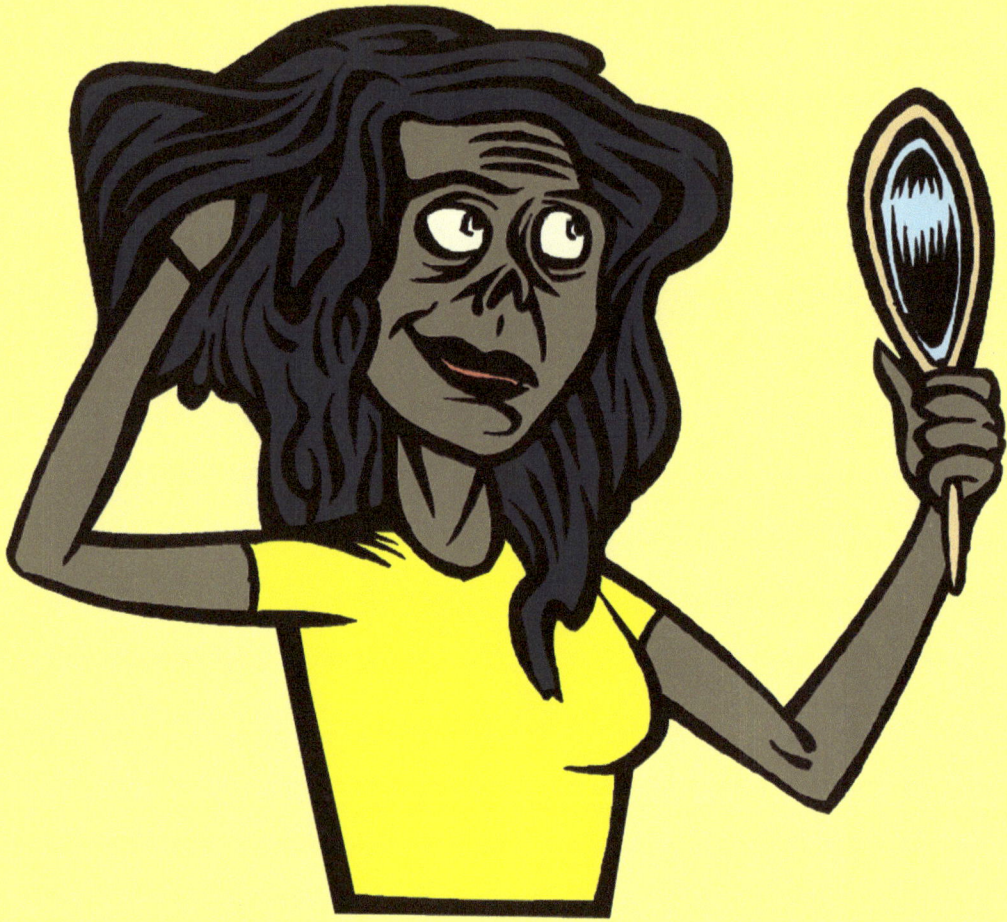

It looked like you.

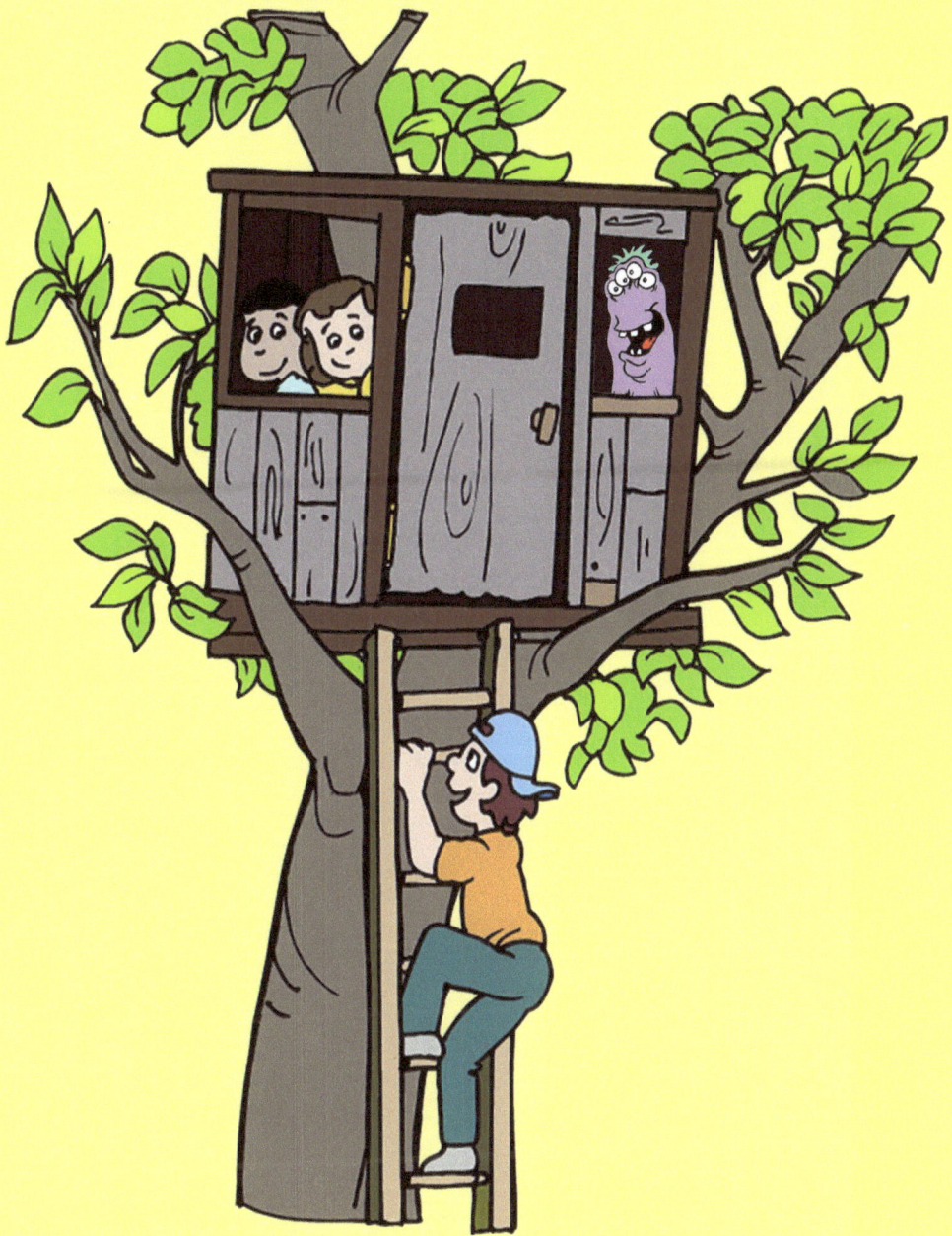

I do not always stay where it is safe.

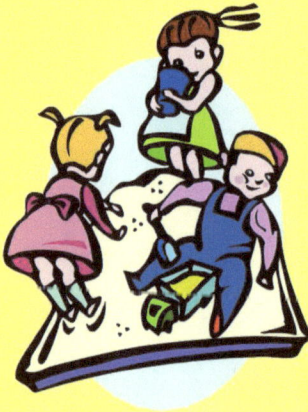

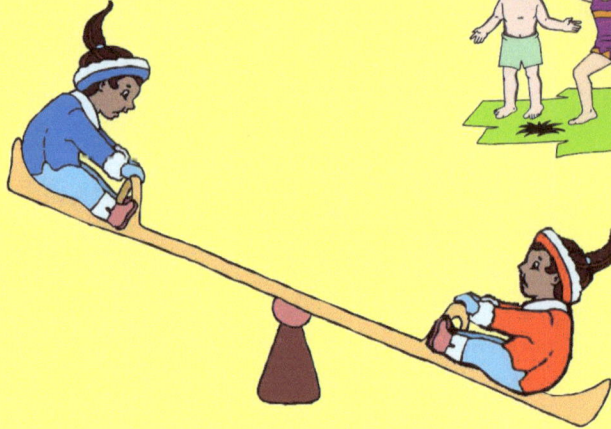

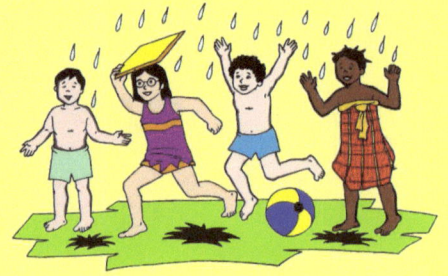

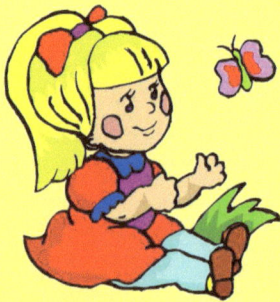

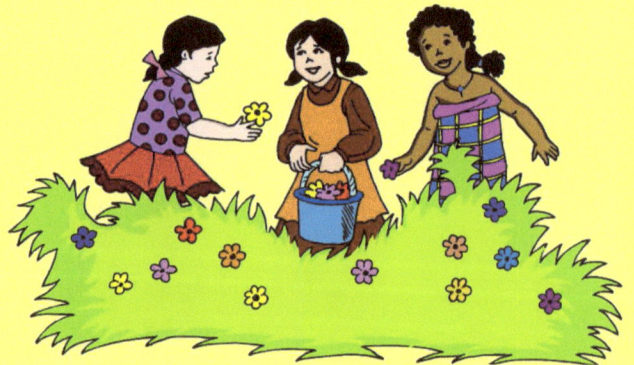

I AM A KID !!!!

And it's not my fault,
what that monster did.

NOT!

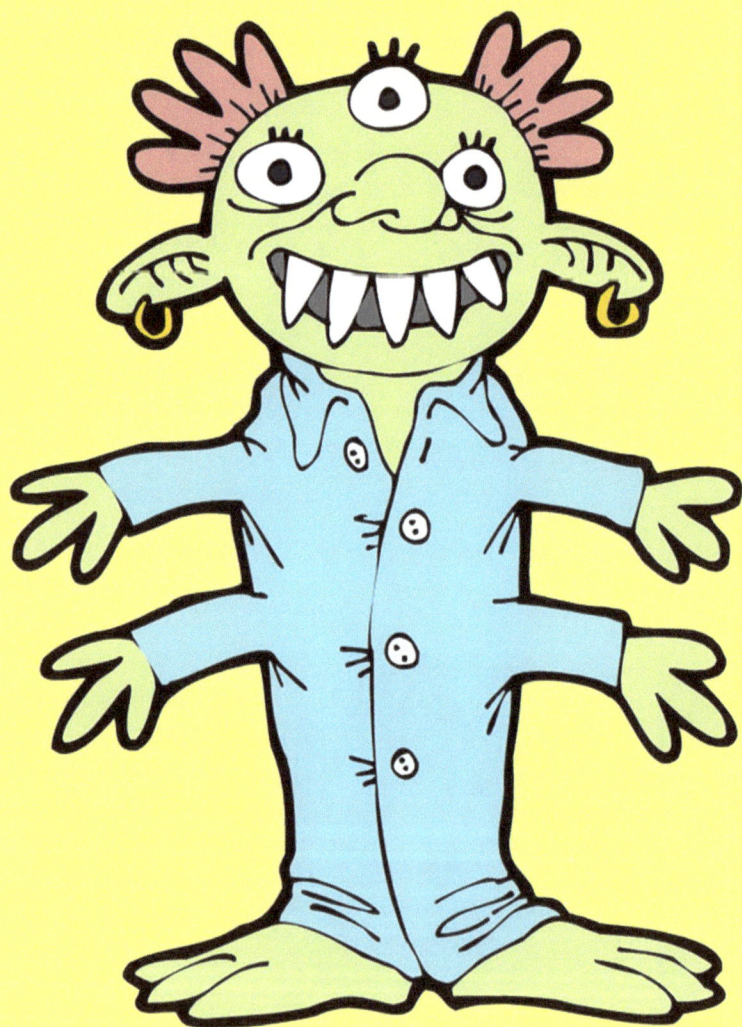

A monster got me this is true.

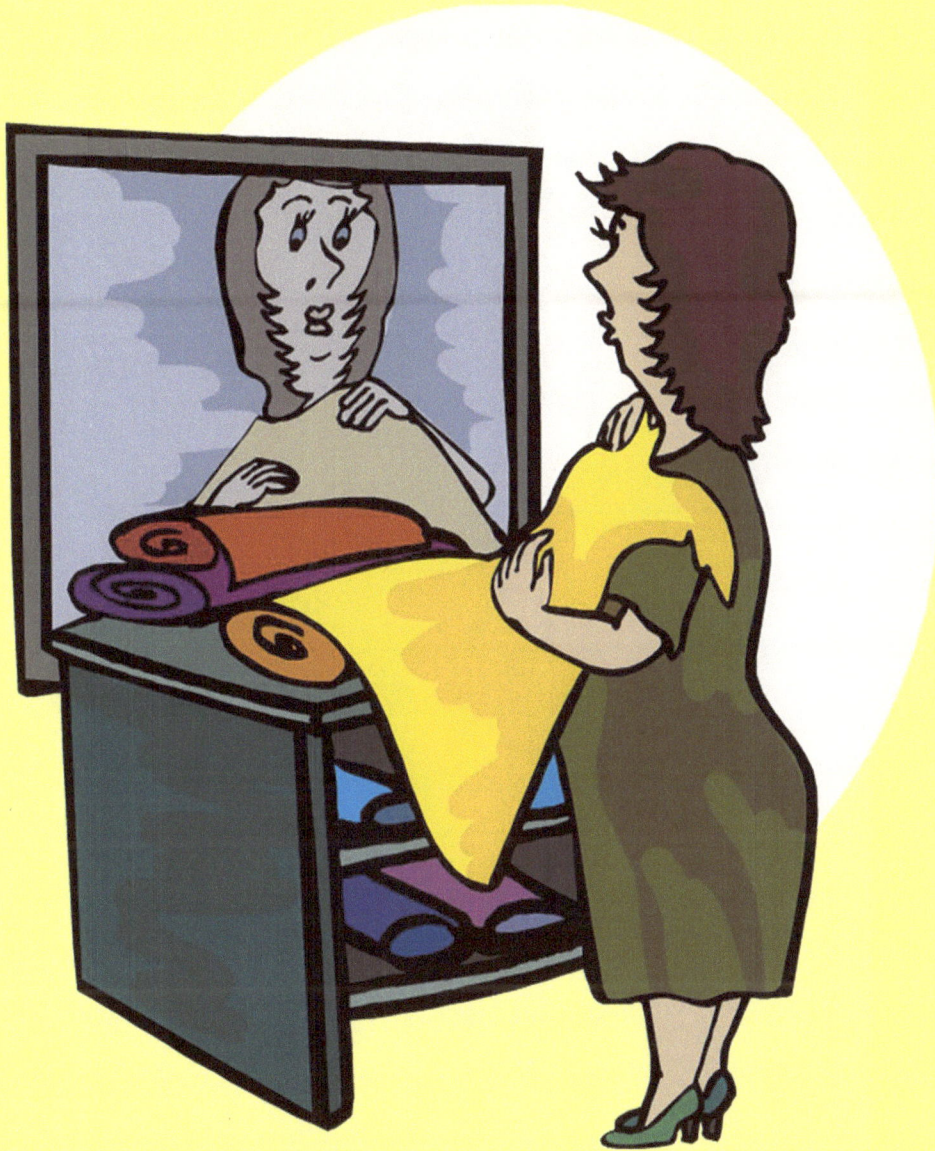

It looked like me.

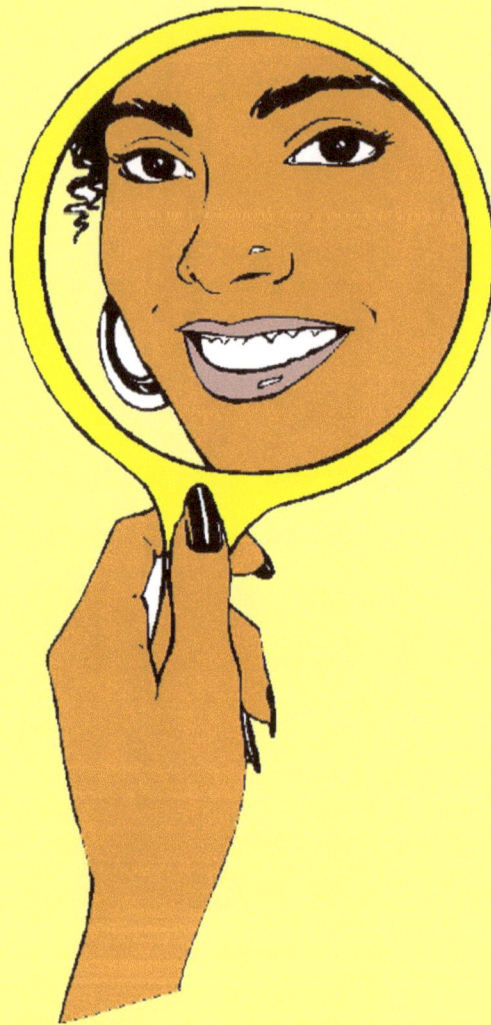

It looked like you.

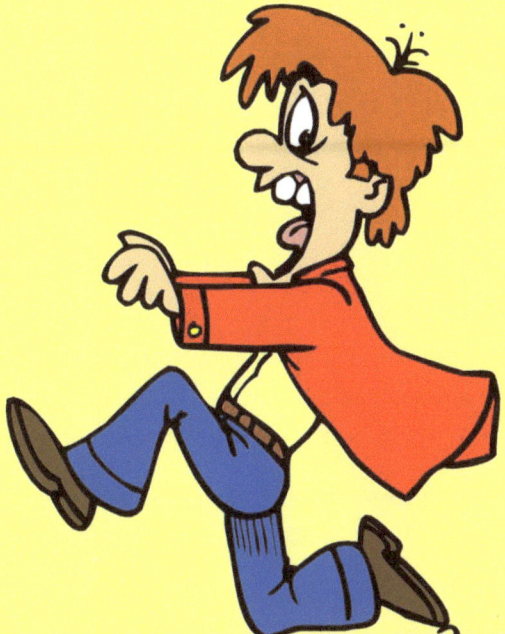

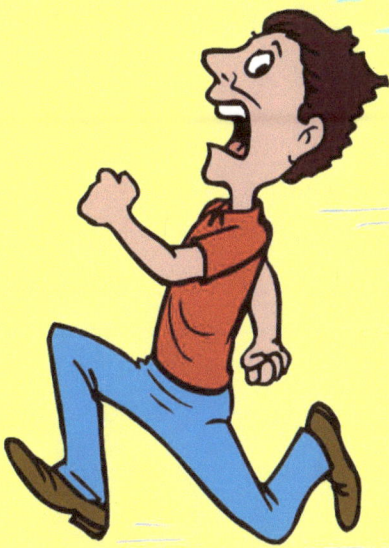

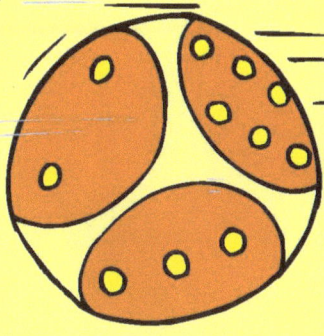

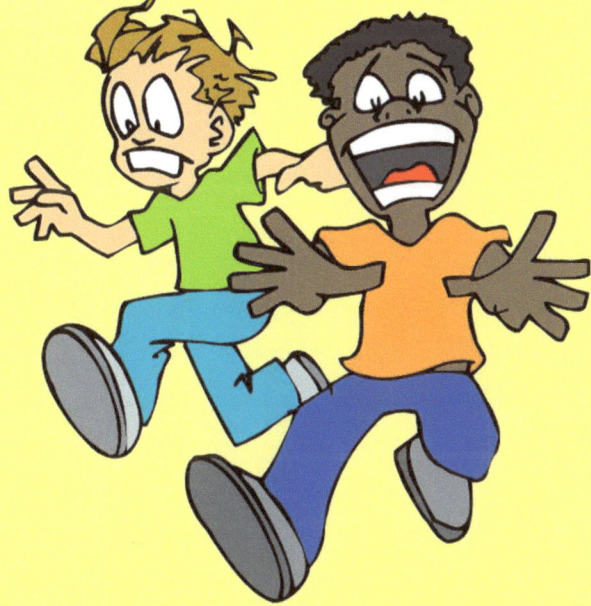

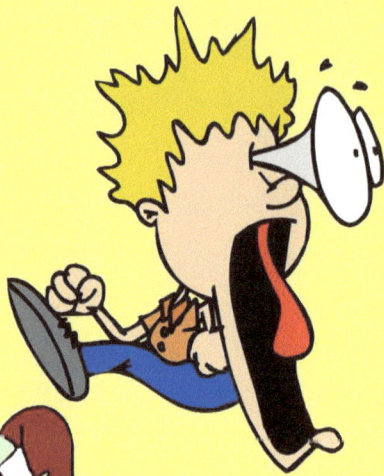

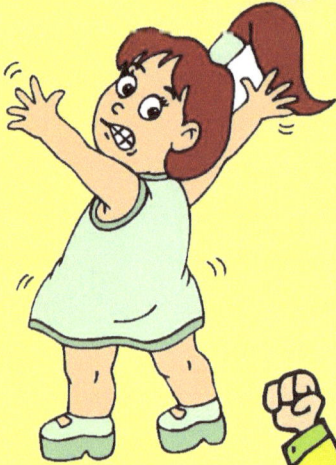

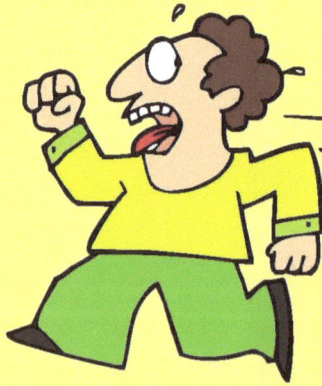

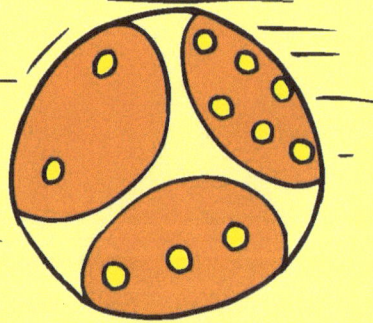

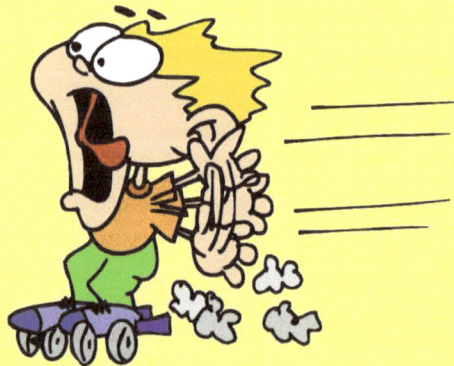

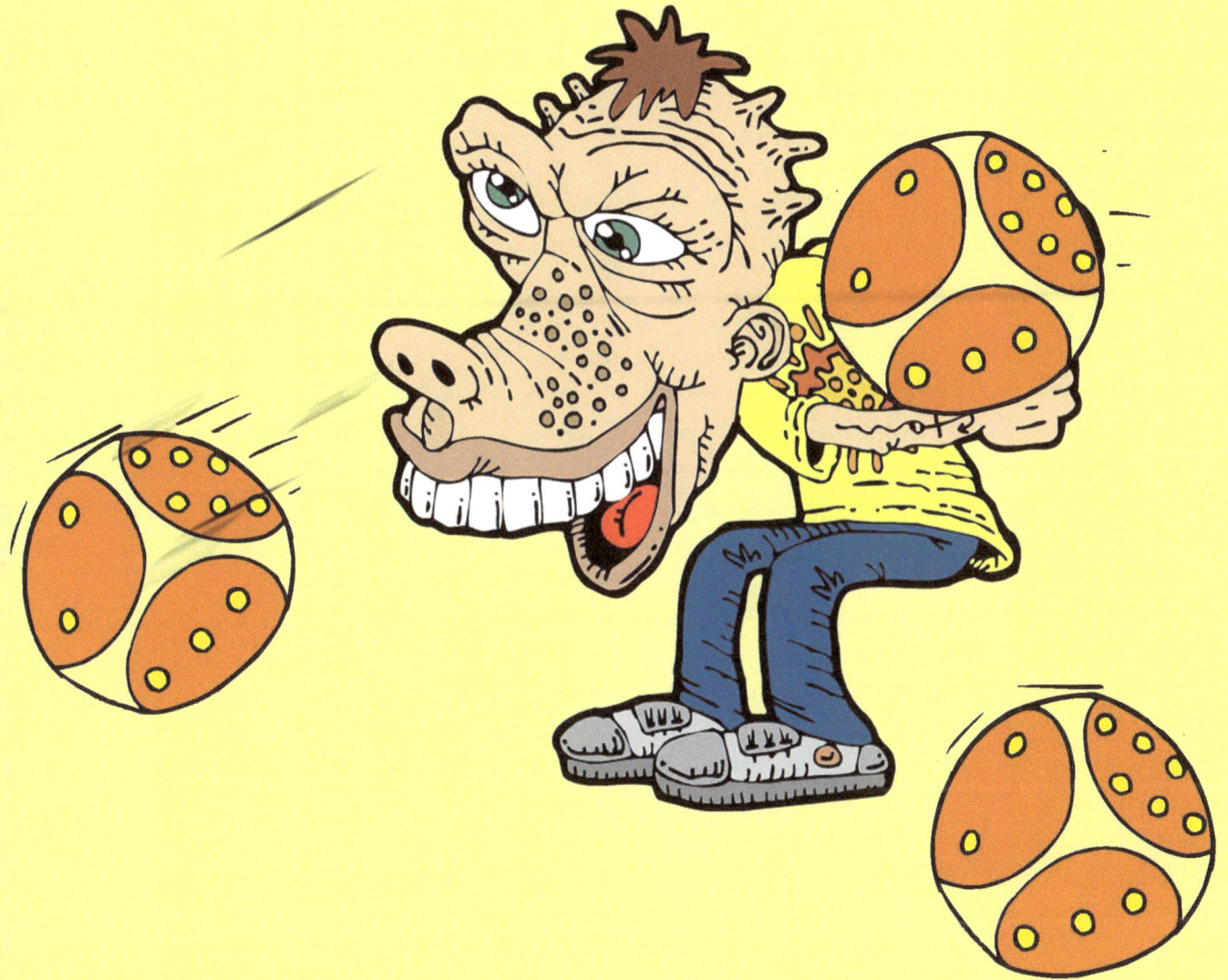

I ran and ran to get away,
but it got me anyway.

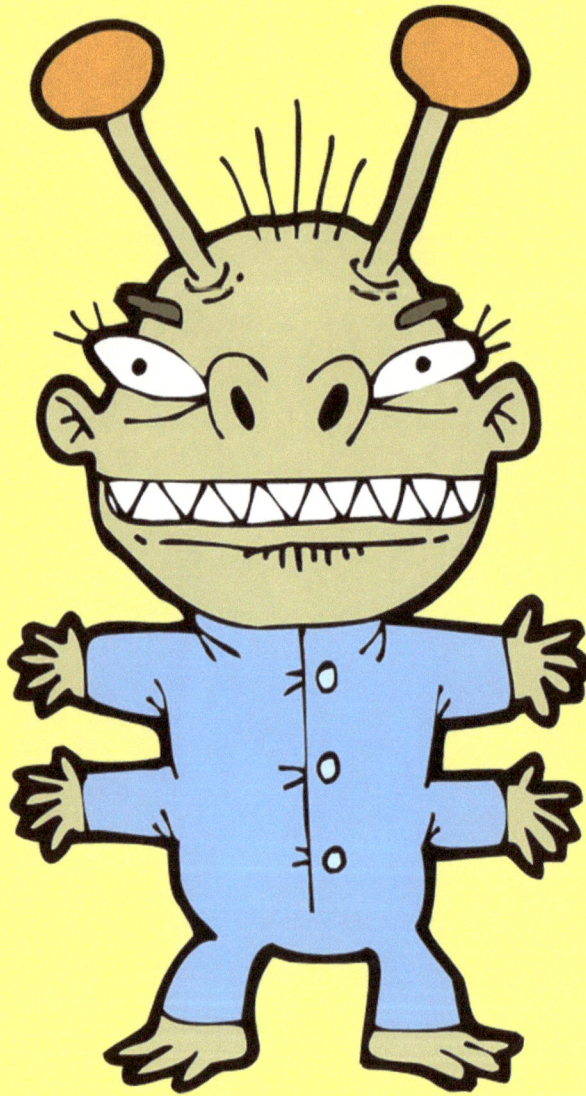

A monster got me this is true.

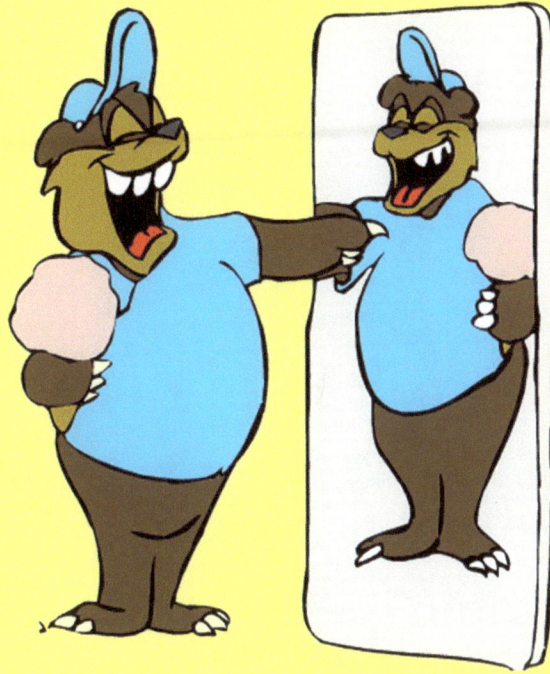

It looked like me.

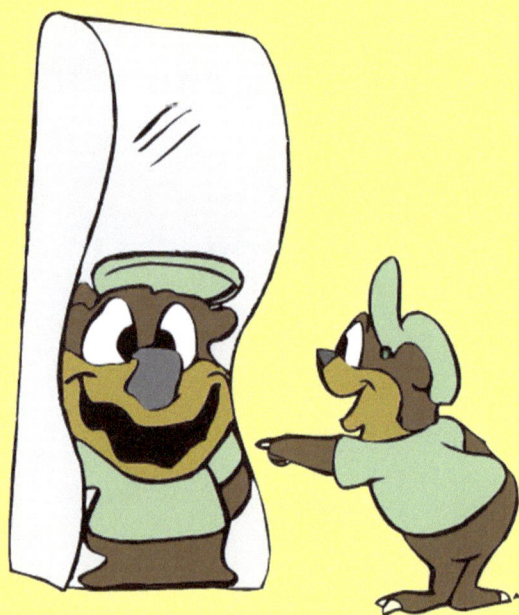

It looked like you.

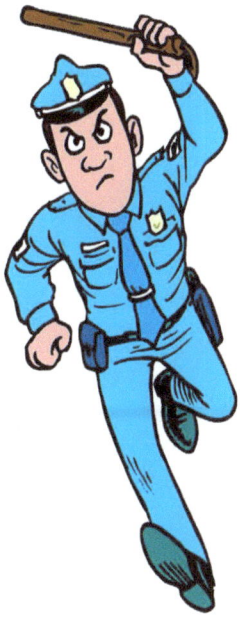

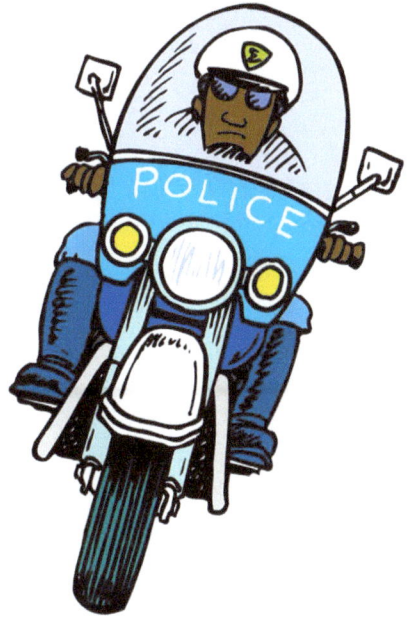

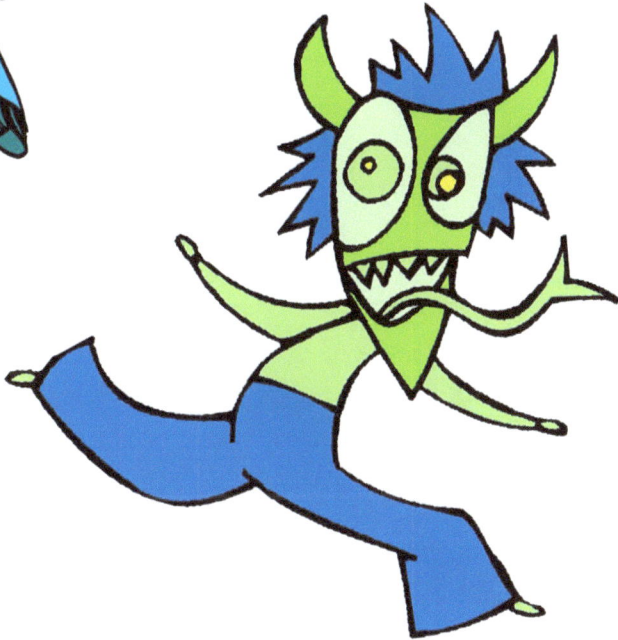

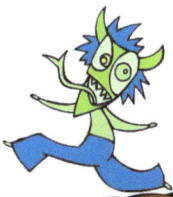

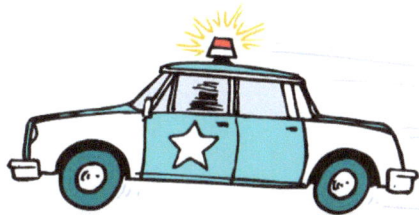

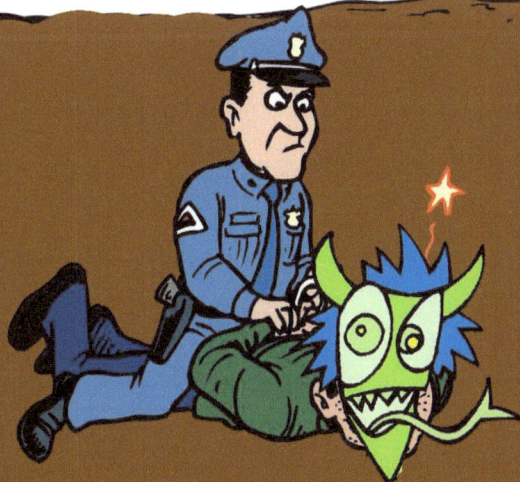

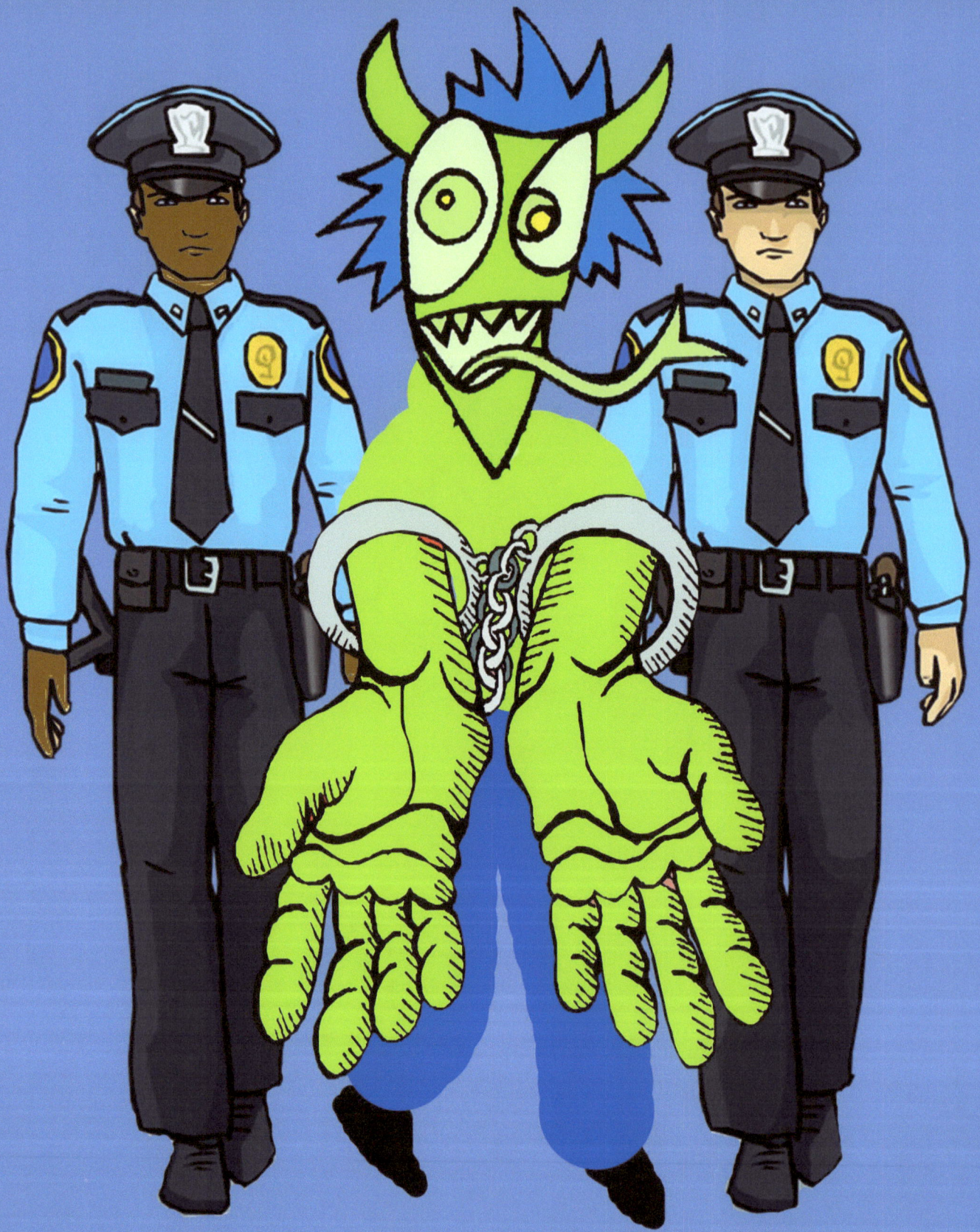

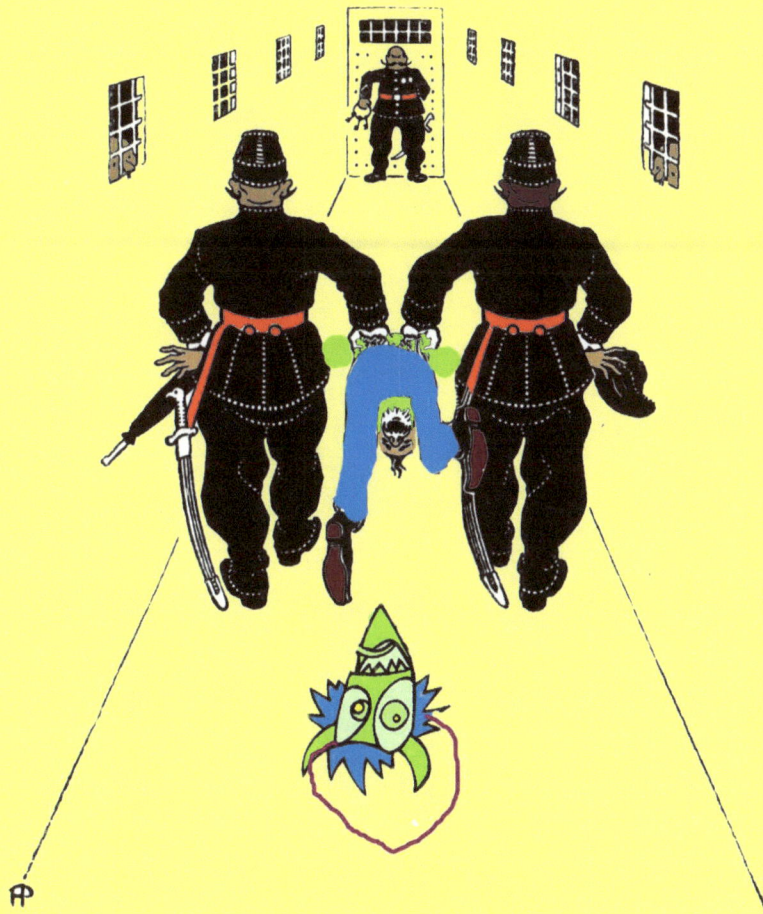

Now I live another day to see that monster put away.

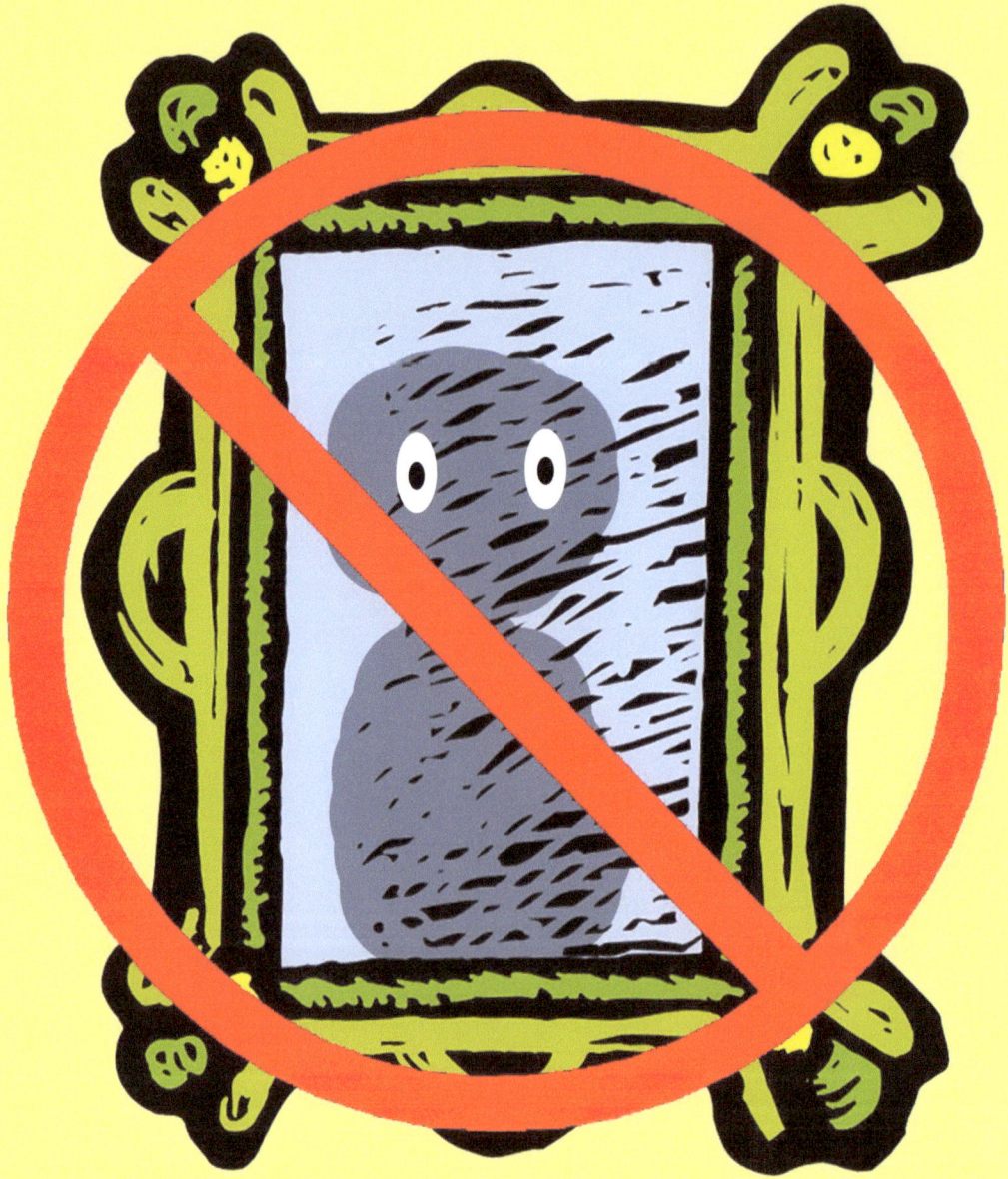

A monster got me this is true, and it's not my fault.

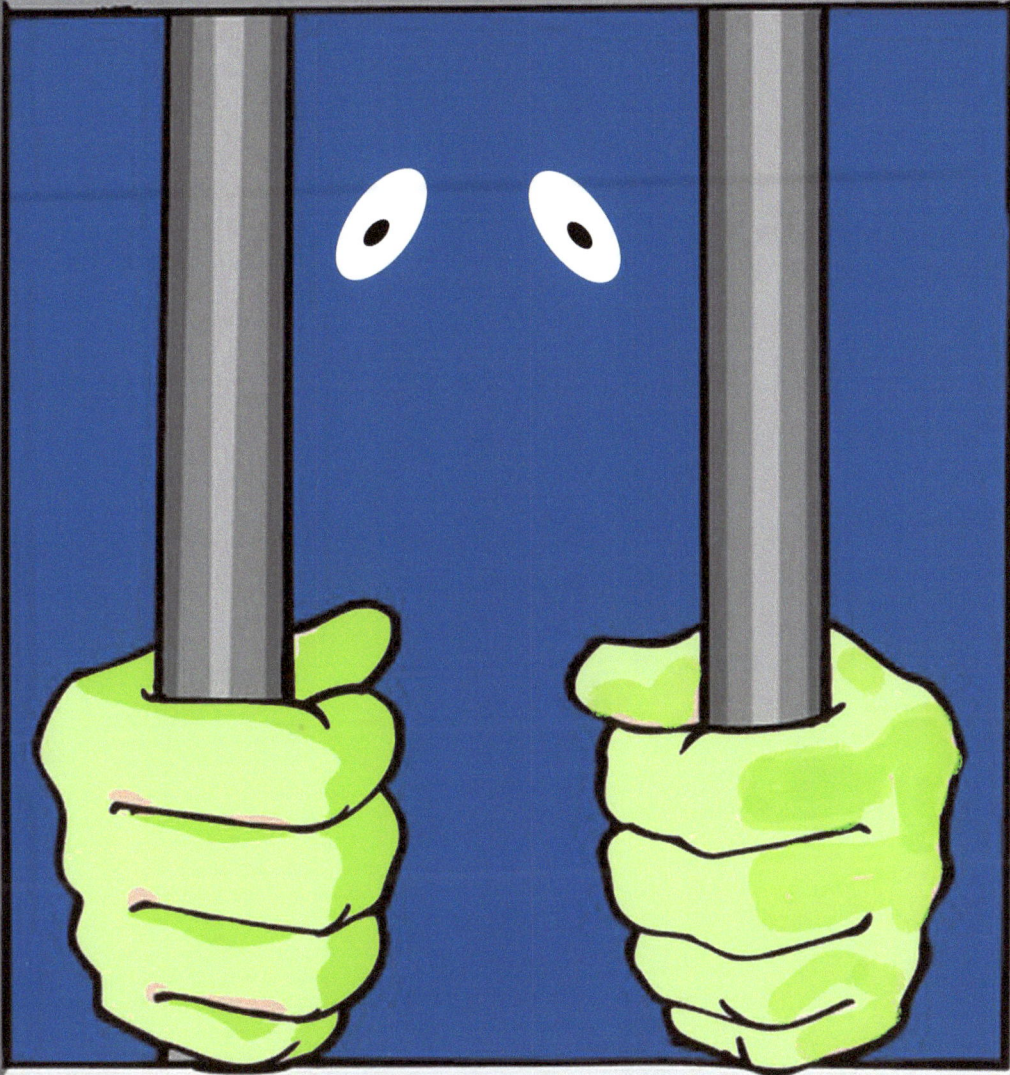

And because I told someone who cared, the monster was caught. Now it can't get you.

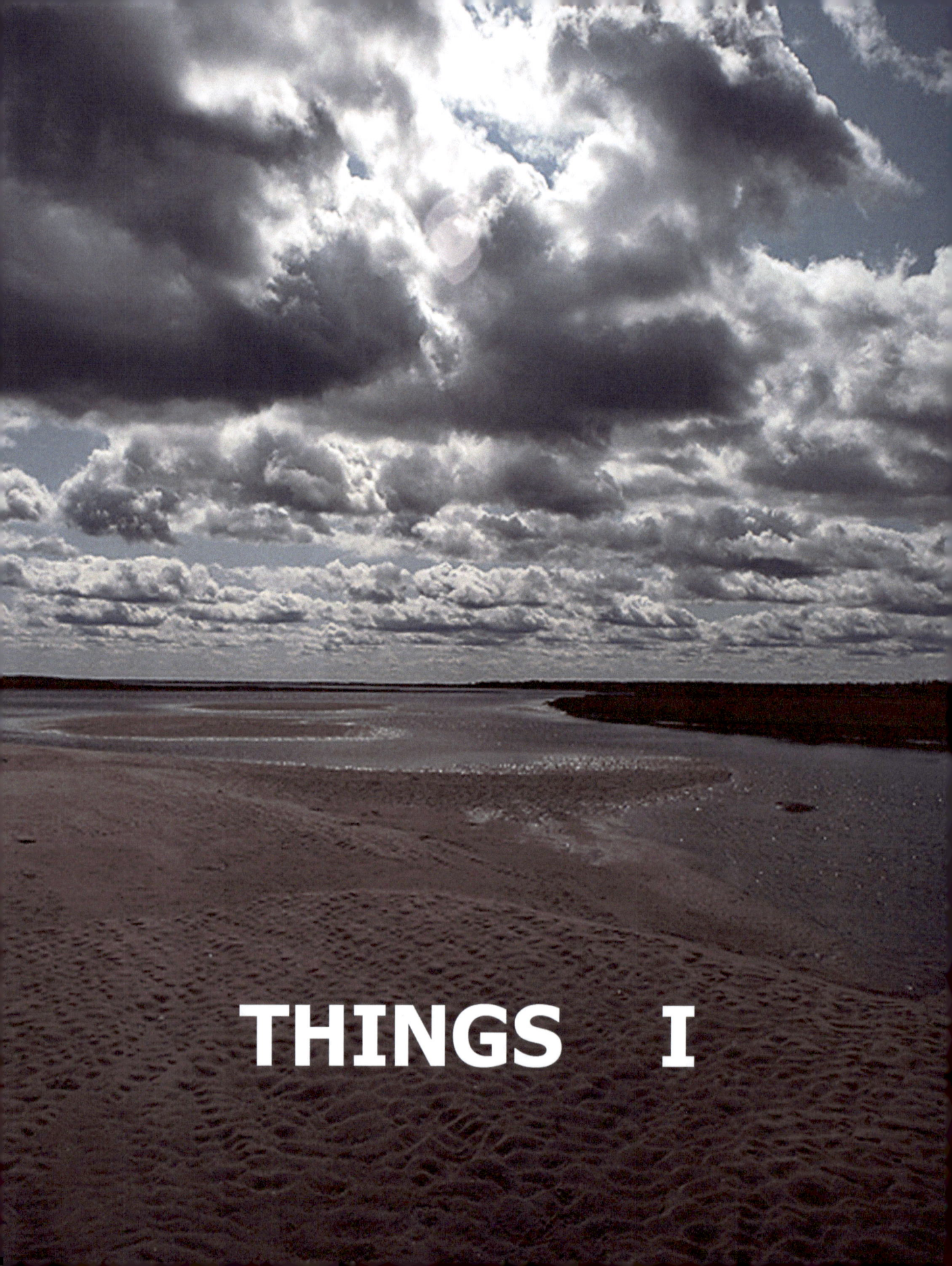

THINGS I

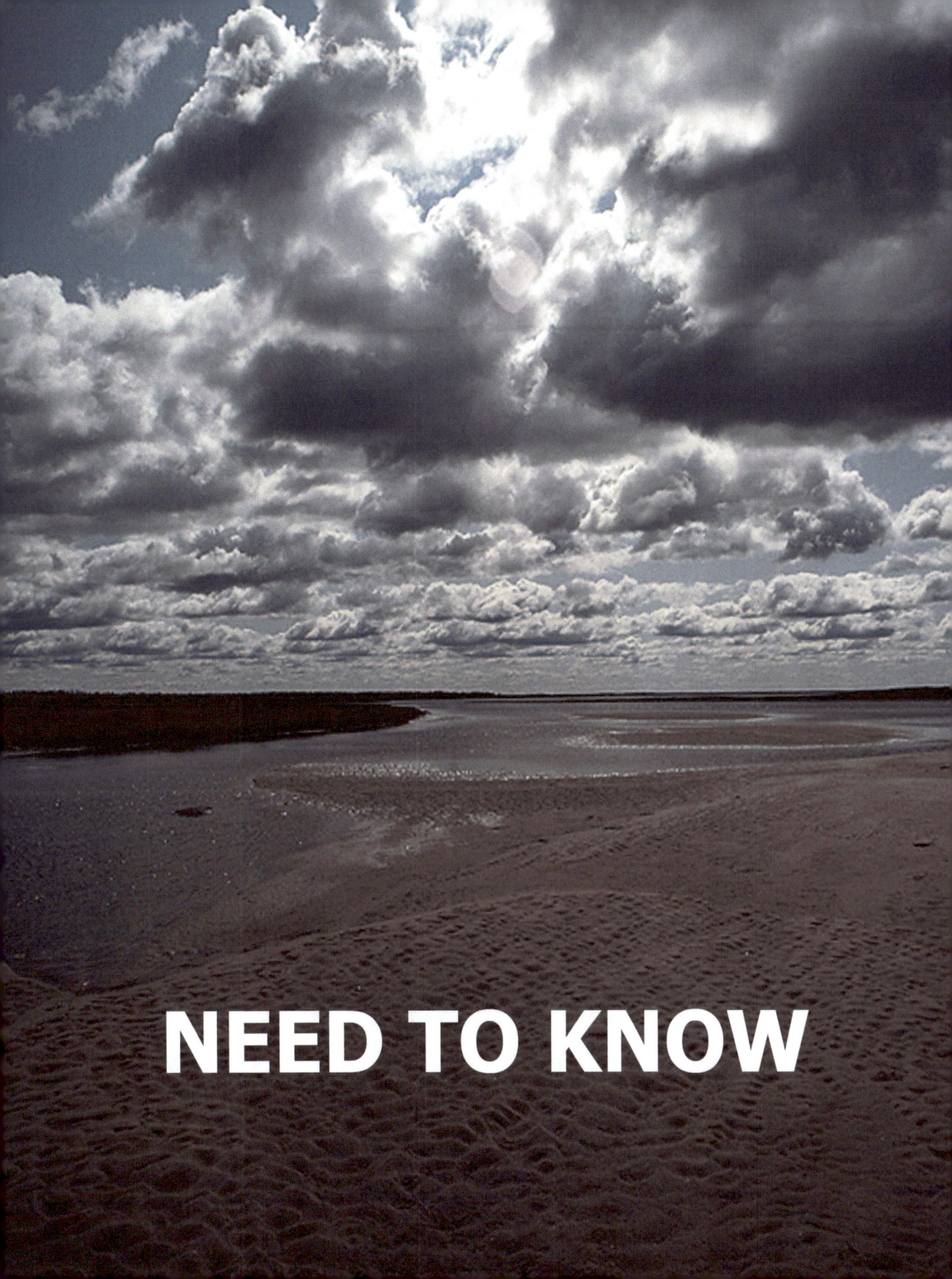

NEED TO KNOW

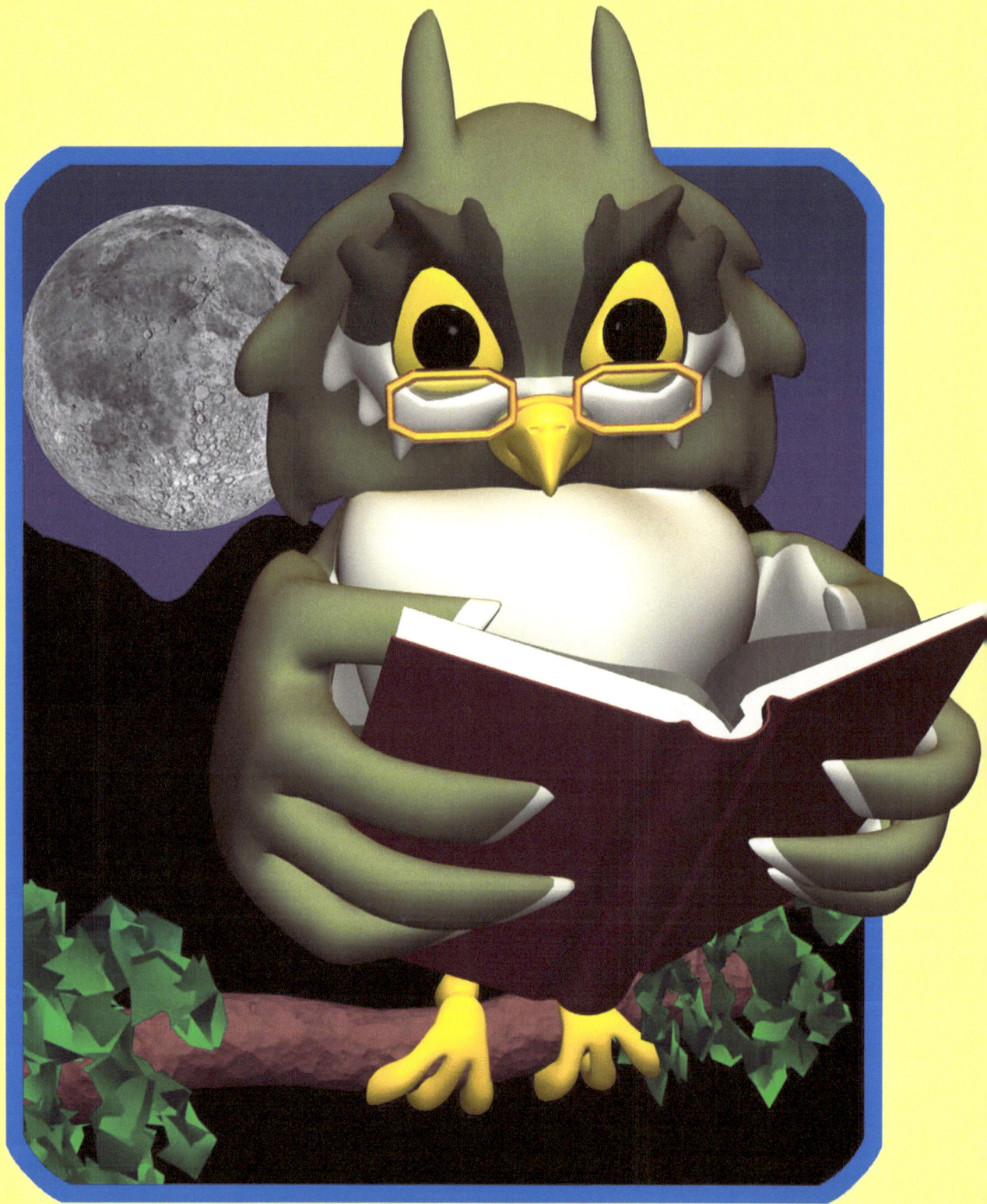

I WILL TREAT MYSELF WELL.

I SHALL BE AWARE OF OTHERS.

NO MEANIES!

I will tell the people who care about me how I feel.

The body heals and renews.

I will let the good in and let the good out.

I will survive.

I am part of everything. Humans are made from the same stuff as the stars.

Everyone needs help.

I will seek help from a higher power.

Be patient things change. I will not always be a kid! Some day I will be an adult.

I will brush my teeth and take a shower or bath every day.

I WILL LISTEN TO THOSE WHO CARE!

I WILL NOT GIVE UP!

I AM GREAT!

BE PATIENT!

DO NOT GIVE UP!

BELIEVE IN YOURSELF

AND

YOUR POWER TO SURVIVE!

I Parent

I'm not perfect, nor are you.
However, I'm here to help you through all of life's steps needed to make you, you.
Sometimes, quite often, I must direct, making sure you do that which is correct.
This is because one day your turn it will be.
I'll help while I can, but life's not forever you'll see.
And by then I hope you will know, of all the things that helped you grow.
At times I may seem tough, angry, and gruff,
But I have little time and so much stuff.
One day you will know how it feels to be me.
And with caring and love I'll hope you'll see, that it is best to use your God given abilities.
One more thing important for you to learn, is respect for yourself is easy to earn.
But first one must avoid the company of fools, and focus on following the rules.
Work hard to find your way by seeking knowledge in books,
and be careful to avoid all of the crooks.
For learning and earning are forever tied, essential to maintain your pride.
And one day, one not too far, you'll be passing along treasures and knowledge, just like I.
So for now stop the scrunching and whining, and do what you're told,
for someday if fortunate you too will find gold, and write such a heart felt poem when you're old.

-Charles J. Stippick

About the Author

I became the foster parent of my (now adopted) son Stephen in December of 2003. I was unaware of the full extent of my son's special needs until a few weeks into the role of Foster Dad. During this time, I began to realize that my son suffered from numerous social and medical disorders that were undiagnosed. This compelled me to seek outside support.

I found that it was impossible to acquire the much needed services as an individual. At the time, doctors who specialized in treating conditions induced by child abuse were few and far between, and those that were within reach, had long waiting lists.

As a result, I began to search for tools that would be helpful for my son, but found very few resources. I eventually found The Camden County Partnership for Children (CCPFC). I acknowledge that the services provided by CCPFC were instrumental to my son's recovery. I urge you as a parent to be proactive. If need be, seek out State and local agencies that specialize in family services and child abuse treatment.

Help is out there, just ask, I did.

Charles Stippick

www.ingramcontent.com/pod-product-compliance
Lightning Source LLC
LaVergne TN
LVHW072119070426
835511LV00002B/27